Keto for Drinkers

How to Eat Keto, Drink, and Still Lose Up to 30 Pounds in 90 Days

ART MAWKIN

Disclaimer: Consult your medical professional prior to going on any diet. Not doing so, could be dangerous to your health. The copyright holder, author, nor the publisher make any medical claims and nothing in this book is intended to take the place of your medical professional.

DEDICATION

To Mark Twain who said:
Take all things in moderation, especially moderation.

.

CONTENTS

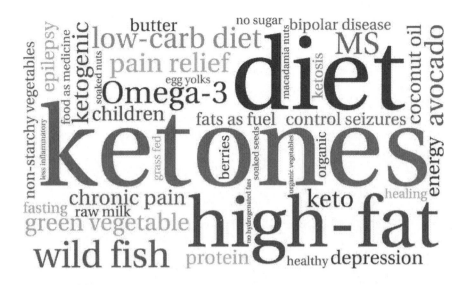

INTRODUCTION
KEEPING IT REAL

There's no such thing as GOOD FOODS and BAD FOODS anymore. It always seemed wrong to attach any moral judgement to specific foods. Just because I enjoy the occasional Swiss Cake Roll, doesn't mean the Little Debbie logo should have her dressed like a hooker. I have a great disdain for all the food-Nazi's who would have us go through a weigh-in and a background check in order to own a knife and a fork. Good food is undeniably one of the great pleasures of life; it doesn't belong on the battleground. So let's just be nice to each other, ok? We put a man on the moon, so there has to be a way to eat great food and enjoy our drinks, too. I know it can be done because I did it. I did it while sitting at a computer most of the day and I never bought any supplements except my morning vitamin. I didn't join a diet plan, join a Google slim-down group, and never ate even one of those frozen diet meals.

Did you ever notice that most diet books are written and sold by either skinny doctors or by women who used to weigh 380 pounds and are now down to 185 - even though they are still only five-foot-two-inches tall?

You are about to learn what I call 'good food math', so get a drink, relax, and read on. As a prelude to Chapter One, I want to give you two of my favorite quotes:

"I drink in order that my friends are more interesting." - Ernest Hemingway

"No good story ever started with someone eating a salad." - Anonymous

CHAPTER 1 HOW TO EAT DRINK AND BE MERRY

Ketosis was a word I had heard but knew little about. My son and daughter-in-law were losing weight rather quickly and they were doing it by eating copious amounts of roasted chicken, steak, and pot roasts. They were excited about their new diet and all the great food they were able to eat. They texted us snapshots of it and featured their diet food in twice-a-week facetime calls. My son said, "Dad, it isn't like I'm pigging-out at every meal, but I can eat just about all the high fat and protein food I want and still lose weight. Immediately, I asked him, "If I was on your diet, could I go down to Shane's (the local BBQ place) and eat a whole rack of ribs? He said, "Sure, I suppose so."

Then I decided to push the envelope; I asked my son, "Can I still drink booze?" My smile turned into a frown when he answered, "Nope, none of that. The diet we are on is like keto but not exactly; it's called the "Whole 30" - and no alcohol is allowed. We are not drinking any beer or drinks while we are on our whole-30. I thought to myself, "I knew it sounded too good to be true. Damn."

3. Alcohol

No alcohol for cooking or drinking is to be consumed while doing Whole30. This includes vanilla extract. You can have something like kombucha, however, which does include a very minor amount of alcohol (as long as there isn't added sugar from outside of fruit juice). Read more about Kombucha restrictions here.

Truth be told: In the above "3. Alcohol," when I saw "This includes vanilla extract." I had to wonder what kind of tight-ass would feel the need to put that in there. The little voice in my head did its Groucho impersonation, "That's the most ridiculous thing I ever heard!". I'm no rocket scientist but I know the alcohol evaporates during cooking - and when most recipes only call for one tiny teaspoon - and you won't be eating a whole pie or cake. No one I ever met has popped a heavy waistline by over indulging via vanilla extract. And "Read more about Kombucha restrictions." WTF?

I looked up Whole-30 to see if it was something I might try, even though I'd have to give up my evening drinks. What I am about to say now is only my personal take on what any diet should or shouldn't be; you have to make up your own mind when it comes to you.

The moment I saw Whole-30 has doctors where you could sign-up, a best-seller book, a giant article in the NEW YORK TIMES, and a group of "whole 30 approved" foods that included a specially made jerky, dressings, collagen enhancers (really!), and so on ----- I thought to myself, "Here we go again. This is everything I hate about diets." The more I read about this diet, the less enthusiastic I became. To me, this "plan" reeked of just one more 'starve your ass off and take it to the gym' hype job. When I see a diet that requires me to carry a book, a calculator, and a bag of energy-bars, my excite-o-meter goes to zero.

I've long suspected that the Universe will eventually punish all co-workers that tell me three times a day, "I got up at 5:30, so I could go to the gym this morning."

A month later, my son -who loves IPA beer- phoned me from a pub and told me they were having beers and wine and their 30-days on "Whole 30" was over and they were celebrating. I silently wondered how much "celebrating" was going to translate into putting weight back on. Eating food to celebrate weight-loss is like having a cigarette to celebrate quitting smoking. They had each lost over 15 pounds in just four weeks. I had to admit, it seems they ate some great food and they lost a lot of weight quickly - and they kept their success by becoming more aware of what they eat.

My theory is that if you are on a diet and you are counting down the days until it's over - you will probably gain most of the weight back.

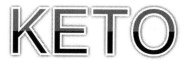

In Case You Live in a Cave

The simple definition of keto, ketogenic is this:

You change your diet to eat the things that will have your body burning fat instead of carbohydrates.

You simply change from:

high-carb / low fat
to
high-fat / low-carb.

There's no such thing as GOOD FOODS and BAD FOODS any more.

How is it different than the widely publicized recommended diet?

Expressed as a percentage of calories of your diet, these are the approximate averages of a range:

Old Way : (Recommended Daily)
55%   Carbs
27% Fat
23% Protein

New Way : (Ketogenic)
6%   Carbs
71 %   Fat
23%   Protein

Even more simply put: Eat 1/10th of the carbs and 3 times more fat, keep protein about the same.

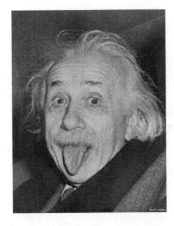

"If you can't explain it to a six year old, you don't understand it yourself."

$^-$ **Albert Einstein**

If you want to do something different from most people you must:

- Think Differently

- Be Willing to Take Criticism from Others

- Do Things Differently

History and Origin

Russel Wilder first used the ketogenic diet to treat epilepsy in 1921. He also coined the term "ketogenic diet." For almost a decade, the ketogenic diet enjoyed a place in the medical world as a therapeutic diet for pediatric epilepsy and was widely used until its popularity ceased with the introduction of antiepileptic agents. The popularity and resurgence of the ketogenic diet as a rapid weight loss formula is a relatively new concept the has shown to be quite effective, at least in the short run.

Things You Won't Have to Do on Keto:

There is no need to announce to anyone you are on a diet.

Once you start dropping the pounds, people will want to know how you are doing it.   Tell them they'll have to change almost everything they think they know about dieting.

You won't need to weigh food, put it in small containers to lug around with you, or obsess about your next meal. You'll be able to eat thousands of good foods and as much as you want.

You won't have to keep a place in your closet for your "fat clothes," the ones you wear between Thanksgiving and the middle or March.

You won't have to lie to your Google Hangout friends doing "The 21 Day Challenge."

You won't have to listen to your physician's speech about how you must start losing weight. The shaming sessions are a thing of the past!

If you want to mess with your doctor's head a little, just say, "I see you've gained a little weight. I think the pounds look good on you but you should be careful not to overdo it of course."

And you won't have to forget how good bacon smells when it's cooking.

CHAPTER 2: A NEW FOOD VIEW

The first thing I did was Google to see how many carbs a day were recommended by a government-backed healthy recommendations. A grown adult of average build can handle about 1500 to 2000 calories a day, and if following healthy guidelines, he/she can eat from 225 to 325 grams of carbohydrates a day. It varies from person-to-person due to size, weight, and life-style (from couch-potato to lumberjack.) Here's one of the top listings that gave me some hope that I could keep drinking my beer or wine while I was on a keto food diet.

So, if you get **2,000 calories** a day, between 900 and 1,300 **calories** should be from **carbohydrates**. That translates to between 225 and 325 grams of **carbohydrates a day**. You can find the carbohydrate content of packaged **foods** on the **Nutrition** Facts label. Feb 7, 2017

Carbohydrates: How carbs fit into a healthy diet - Mayo Clinic
https://www.mayoclinic.org/healthy.../nutrition-and...eating/.../carbohydrates/art-200457...

Like most people, I could not visualize what a plate of food that has "between 225 and 325 grams of carb" would look like. As soon as I saw this Google listing, my very next act was to Google to see "how many carbs a day on the ketogenic diet?" My logic was simple: I wanted to see how a plate of 'regular meal' and a 'keto meal' would compare. I already knew what I would do after that; I'd see how many carbs are in the drinks I like - and then check to see how many I could squeeze into my day. "How many drinks I can squeeze into a day," is not a phrase that is ever going to roll off the lips of your doctor.

So here's what I found when I Googled: How many carbs a day are allowed in the ketogenic diet?

If I'm honest, I have to tell you the first result I read was written by a doctor and it recommended "that 20 grams a day" maximum carbs "would be low enough to put almost anyone into ketosis." I didn't like this answer; it sounded like something most doctors would say if there was a lawyer in the room. So I Googled again and found something I felt was exciting:

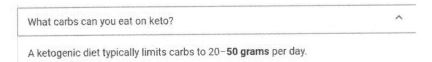

This just confirmed what I always have suspected about most doctors' advice on weight and diet goals: They know you are going to cheat, so if you weigh 200 pounds, they suggest 165, and then - when you get to 185, they reluctantly say, "You are doing ok, so you need to stick with it."

When I saw that wide range of 20 to 50 grams of carbs a day, I decided to cut myself some slack and see what I could do with a number from 30 to 40 carb grams a day. In most of what I read, the doctors gave the lowest figures but many people who had actually lost weight and many dieticians were a little more lenient. I like people who are a little more lenient. I fit into that category.

After I read this, I immediately ran to the pantry and grabbed my loaf of Wonder Bread and read the nutritional label:

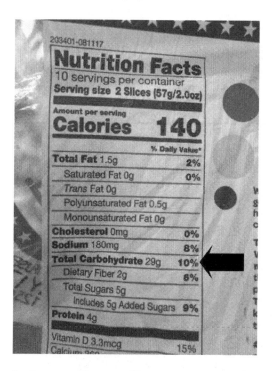

Just so you know: From now on you can skip past the **Calories** on the **Nutrition Facts** and go straight to the **Total Carbohydrate** line.

When I saw that just two slices of WB was 29g of carbs, I thought "Holy Moly! I am free. A diet I can handle." I imagined that between those two slices would be a half-rack of ribs. Here's why: I Googled for "carbs in half-rack of BBQ ribs," and here's what I found.

> Carbohydrates. Meat tends to be very low in **carbohydrates**, and half racks of **ribs** are no exception. Each half rack of **ribs** provides just 2 grams of **carbohydrates**, with no fiber.

In an instant, I thought, I am going to love this diet. I can eat a half rack of ribs between two slices of Wonder Bread, and eat the other half-rack without bread for desert. Even if I allowed myself 40g of carbs a day, I'd still have 11g to go. That's enough for four Michelob Ultras. Quality of life is all about priorities.

Of course, the very next thing, I got back on Google to find the most desirable delicious 11 grams possible.

Voila!

How many carbs does a fried chicken breast have?		
How many calories in Batter-dipped & Fried Chicken Breast, with skin		
(?) **Nutrition Facts**		
Sodium	311mg	13%
Total Carbs. help	10.2g	3%
Dietary Fiber help	0.3g	1%
Sugars help	0g	

If my doctor had just said to me, "Art, I am going to put you on a diet and you can eat a rack of ribs on Wonder Bread, and have a delicious fried chicken (skin on, battered) breast for desert," I would have shouted, "Sign me up now!"

Over my first 90-days, I actually did have a few meals like this and I still stayed on the diet. Most times, I eat a more balanced meal. For example, I can grill a 12-ounce ribeye (0g), four ounces of squash and onions (4 x 1.7 g)= 6.8g, 2 ounces of cheddar cheese (1.0g), one cup of turnips or spinach boiled w/ham bits and all the butter I want, only 7.9g. Grand Total for this meal: 15.7 grams, about half of my daily carb amounts for this great delicious meal.

On most of the diets I ever tried, I was more or less forced to think of "what I can't eat" instead of "what I CAN eat." This difference in the way we are thinking is huge! This is the magic that will help you stay on the keto diet. No other diet I've ever seen offers this.

I love patty sausage and scrambled eggs with lots of cheese. Sausage and cheese eggs have almost zero carbs! I mean a big plate only has 2 or 3 carbs tops! Two eggs with cheese is only 1g of carbs! In my mind, they are FREE.

Welcome to my world: You can eat all the ribeye steaks you want. It takes zero effort to plan a meal if you start with a ribeye. Just one or two sides of vegetables and you're done.

FreshDirect Ribeye Steak   ×

Nutrition Facts

Serving Size   4   oz ↻

Amount Per Serving
Calories   170

% Daily Value*

Total Fat 7g	11%
Saturated Fat 2.5g	13%
Trans Fat 0g	
Cholesterol 79mg	26%
Sodium 62mg	3%
Total Carbohydrate 0g	0%
Dietary Fiber 0g	0%
Sugars 0g	
Protein 26g	
Vitamin A 0 IU	0%
Vitamin C 0mg	0%
Calcium 0mg	0%
Iron 2.2mg	12%

Ribeye Steak

zero ◄

* The % Daily Value (DV) tells you how much a nutrient in a serving of food contributes to a daily diet. 2,000 calories a day is used for general nutrition advice.

If you are going to change the way you eat and get healthier, I have great news for you. Make yourself a grilled or pan-fried ribeye and some zucchini or spicy green beans and top it off with a couple of glasses of wine.

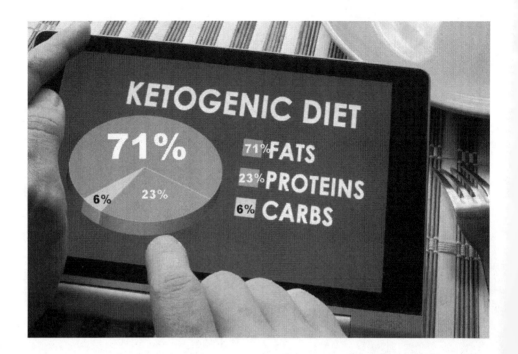

CHAPTER 3: THE NO DIET DIET

An article recently published was headlined:
7 Ways Comfortable Ways to Order in Restaurants When You are on Keto Diet

This is definitely a first-world problem. On our planet, half the world goes to bed hungry - and we have the luxury of going to dinner with friends - and we have to listen to some vegan at the table whining about what they can and cannot eat. One of the greatest things about being on keto is that, unless you are dining out at an ice cream parlor, there is always good stuff to eat.

Let's face the truth here. The most difficult thing about eating in a more healthy way is to get your head adjusted to a new way to think about good food and drink.

The one thing that opened my eyes to what I could do on a keto diet is a baked potato. I love baked potatoes, so the first thing I did was to Google "how many carbs in a baked potato?" Here's the answer:

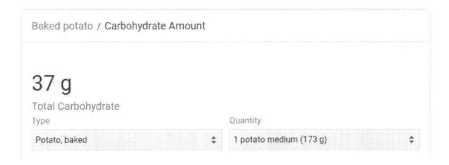

Baked potato / Carbohydrate Amount

37 g
Total Carbohydrate

Type	Quantity
Potato, baked	1 potato medium (173 g)

Since I promised myself to keep my max carbs per day to about 30 to 40g, it only takes one medium baked potato and I'm maxed out. Remember, a man's 2000 calorie a day diet would normally have about 325g of carbs, a woman's 1500 calorie a day would consist of about 225g. So I'm going all the way down to only 30 to 40 carbs a day, including my drinks. This is a huge difference!

Common sense comes into play here: If I'm dropping from 325g down to no more than 30 to 40 g/day, then whether I have 27 or 42g on any given day is a very small difference.

There is such a thing as "the law of diminishing returns." My taking in 27 to 42 grams of carbs is only a difference of 27/325 = 8.3% to 42/325 = 12.9%. This means I'm reducing my carbs by 92% to 87%, so long as I'm in that range. That is tremendous progress. If I stay around 90%, I am going to lose weight. A doctor or do-gooder blog-writing soccer mom are not going to cut you any slack at all, but you'll be doing absolutely great! The numbers don't lie.

There is so much misinformation out there. Just because you have an extra 4 g of carbs one day doesn't drop you out of ketosis and send you all the way back to the starting line. That's ridiculous. Such statements are guilt-shaming rhetoric spread by people who are bad at math. Shaming might work on a 4-year-old, but hey - we are all adults here.

I have a cousin who has been losing weight for years, just not every year. What he does is very effective and smart. Years ago, he said to me, "When I want to lose some weight, I just quit eating everything that is white." I realize now, he's a genius. That is the perfect way to define the keto diet. No sugar, bread, potatoes, milk, grits. I guess egg whites and white wine would be the exceptions.

I want to explain to you why I consider the lowly baked potato as my personal gateway to the keto diet. Right after I found that a medium baked potato has 37 grams of carbs, I Googled again. I had just switched to drinking a low carb beer, one of the lowest at only 2.6 grams per 12 ounces, Michelob Ultra. It blew me away when I divided 37 by 2.6 and got = 14.2   That's how many beers I could drink a day and still stay on my keto diet. Let me hasten to add, I didn't plan on drinking 14 beers a day - or eating a baked potato a day. But this was the moment it hit me, what a great tradeoff I had found. No way I wanted to stop drinking but I suddenly realized that keto offered me a compromise that I found totally acceptable.

More or less, I can drink all the beer I want each day AND I can eat as many ribeye's, pork chops, fried chicken, and limited veggies as I want. I am an experienced drinker and I know for a fact that my few drinks at day's end reduces my appetite, so it just seemed to me that this kind of keto was the kind that just might agree with me. Plus, over the next three months I dropped just over 30 pounds - and if I'm honest I had about two or three 'cheat days' per month along the way.

I had already cut down sugar years ago by using Splenda, and except for couple of deserts per month, I hardly eat the white stuff anymore anyway. In fact, I went to a restaurant and the waitress brought me one of those Southern double-sweet iced teas with lemon. I drank it and had the worse feeling, just a dull bloated "I should-not-have-eaten-that feeling." That was my body telling me I was doing fine without all the sugar.

How many calories in Little Debbie Creme Pies, Oatmeal

	(?) Nutrition Facts	
Cholesterol help	0mg	0%
Sodium	190mg	8%
Total Carbs. help	26g	9%
Dietary Fiber help	0.5g	2%

CHAPTER 4: NEW FOOD MATH

1 oatmeal cream pie = 10 Michelob Ultra Beers
Skip the Little Debbie and have a beer or glass of wine instead.

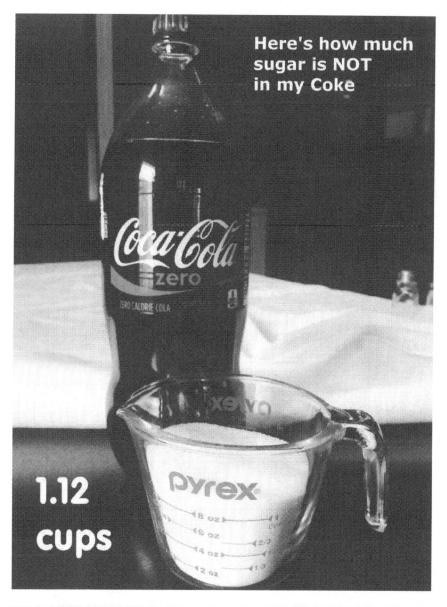

When I discovered I can drink all the beers, wine, or spirits I wanted and all I had to give up was bread and potatoes, it became easy for me to stay on keto. Whenever I wanted a piece of cake or a candy bar, I just drank a beer instead. I can't ever imagine anyone giving me advice like that, but it just seemed so right somehow to me.

In only three months, I lost five inches off my waist. My love-handles were half the size, and my underwear didn't fit any more. All the while I was eating ribeye's, having dinner of BBQ pork and vegetables, and drinking all the 2.6 carb beer I wanted.

After the first six weeks, I was into the last notch on my belt and I hardly felt like I was getting started. The greatest surprise of all was yet to come: I was actually eating less and less each week simply because my food cravings were dropping off. I never expected this to happen but it makes perfect sense. My body was getting really great food and I was able to eat most of my favorite things. And by golly, I was able to keep drinking.

To be honest with you, I have to tell you about an adjustment I did have to make. I had been drinking mostly Budweiser regular beer for years. It is about 4.82% ABV (alcohol by volume.) The Michelob Ultra I switched to is 4.20%.

So the buzz-factor in terms of alcohol content was reduced by about 12.8%. I love math. This means if I had been drinking 6 beers a day, I'd have to drink 6.77 beers a day to get the same buzz. I thought to myself, "Hell one more beer a day; I can do it!" Now, that some math your doctor will *never* do for you.

Actually I average about 4 beers a day, so I'd only have to drink about an extra half beer a day to keep up my regular buzz. I felt this was very doable.

I'm telling you stuff here that you will never hear from your doctor or any of your tree-hugging vegan cousins.

I read a line once, it was by D. H. Lawrence, it went like this:

"I never saw a wild thing sorry for itself. A small bird will drop frozen dead from a bough without ever having felt sorry for itself."

Self-pity is unique to human beings; it doesn't exist in Nature. The same can be said for guilt. If a wild animal makes a mistake, they suffer the immediate consequences and it's over. *The human is the only animal that punishes itself over and over again for the same mistake.* If you are going to be on any diet, this is something you should put to memory. You are going to have to lighten up and enjoy the journey. If you feel like celebrating, don't reach for a donut, just pour yourself a drink.

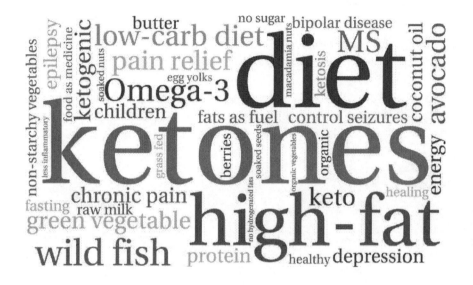

CHAPTER 5: THE 33 STORY BUILDING

The human brain has tremendous powers. We meet thousands of people and know the faces of hundreds of movie stars and our grey matter remembers and sorts those thousands of different facial patterns and rarely ever confuses one with another. It's amazing! Our powers for visual memory are practically unlimited. On the other hand, we can forget a phone number or a name so very easily. Genetics and evolution have formed humans to have a super power of visual memory. Here how I recommend you visualize your keto diet. This is easy to remember and makes perfect sense. Just think of a 33 story building.

Here's what you need to know: A grown man eating a nominal 2000 calorie a day diet takes in a recommended 325 grams of carbs a day. Just think of the 325 grams as a 33 story building. Now when you go to keto - you are only going to eat 30 to 40 grams of carbs a day. Just think of that 33 story building and pretend you now live only on floors 1,2,3,4. As long as you don't go any higher than the 3rd or 4th story, you'll be on keto and losing weight.

Switching from 325 grams to below 30 or 40 is when you start eating fat instead of carbs. Your body will start burning fat instead of carbs as you lose weight and get healthier.

You may have a day or two a month where you only live on floors 1 and 2, and you'll have days you live floor 3 or 4 - and it's ok, you will be just fine.

Your body won't go from keto to zero and you have to start all over from scratch, just because of a very few carbs. If you are going to cheat all the time, you won't succeed, but it's ok to fluctuate just a little from day to day.

How do I know my body is in keto?

If you've been eating less than 30g of carbs for a week, you are there. If you want proof, order you a bottle of urine strip tests. You pee on the strip and wait 30 seconds and the color of the strip will tell you approximately what stage of keto you are in. These urine strips are not extremely accurate, certainly not as accurate as a blood test, but they get the job done. Don't live or die based on these little strips, they are just a quick approximate test for people to buy for the price of a bottle of wine or a six-pack. You clothes not fitting so tight is a better and cheaper 'keto test' in my opinion.

Here's a totally free way to tell if you are in ketosis. Say it's been a week and you stayed below 35 g a day of carbs. Get a tiny pinch of bread, soft bread and place it on the tip of your tongue. If it tastes as sweet as sugar, you are in keto. If it just tastes like regular bread, you've been cheating. When you are in ketosis, your body is ready to convert that carb to sugar in a hurry. If you are in ketosis, it will take less than five seconds for you taste sugar; this works very fast.

Doesn't the alcohol I drink make me backtrack on my keto?

Not as much as you think. Your body will burn the alcohol before getting to the fat somewhat, but those drinks will NOT suddenly throw you out of keto, not at all. It's more of a temporary slowdown, but one most people can easily handle. Keto is not like a binary switch that turns all the lights 'on' and 'off' suddenly. The self-appointed keto cops would have you believe you've suffered fatal damage and have to start-over - when you take a drink, but this just isn't true. The 'keto-cops' will argue this with you all day long; just ignore them and stay on your plan. You'll be fine and when over time when you step on your scales, you will get all the proof you need.

This is just common sense really. You are living on the bottom four floors of a 33 story building and you are not even close to living back up on floor 33 - and eating 325 g of carbs a day - as you used to do. Relax, have a drink.

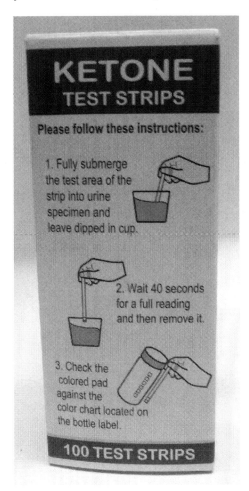

A box of Ketone test strips are a little expensive, especially since once opened they expire in only two months. There are about 50 in a box. I never used mine but twice after a week on the diet and by then I was already losing weight, so didn't find them useful. The little bit of money you spent in buying this book was a better investment.

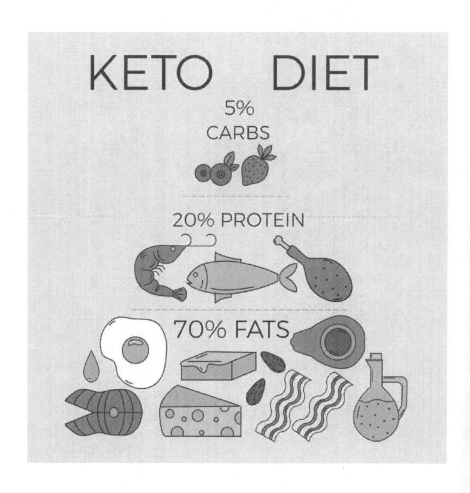

CHAPTER 6: ALCOHOL

Beer Carbs

Beer	ABV	Carbs
Bud Light Platinum	6.0%	4.40
Miller Lite	4.2%	3.20
Michelob Ultra	4.2%	2.60
Miller 64	2.8%	2.40
Bud Select 55	2.4%	1.90
Budweiser Select	4.3%	3.10
Bud Light	4.2%	6.60
Busch Light	4.1%	3.20
Michelob Ultra Amber	4.0%	3.20
Michelob ULTRA Lime Cactus	4.0%	5.50
Milwaukee's Best Light	4.1%	3.50
Natural Light	4.2%	3.20
Corona Light	4.1%	5.00
Coors Light	4.2%	5.00
Keystone Premium	4.4%	5.80
Bud Ice	5.5%	4.00
Leinenkugel"s Light	4.2%	5.70
Grolsch Light Lager	3.6%	6.00
Busch	6.90%	10.20
Heineken	5.00%	11.00
Corona	4.50%	13.00
Corona Extra	4.60%	14.00
Budweiser	5.00%	10.60

Wine Carbs

Wine	ABV	Carbs
Rosé	14.5%	3.00
Sauvingnon Blanc	13.3%	2.50
Burgundy	12.5%	5.50
Sangria	10.0%	3.20
Chardonnay	14.4%	3.00
Skinnygirl White or Red	12.0%	5.00
Merlot	12.5%	3.69
Martini & Rossi Extra Dry	18.0%	5.00
White Zinfandel	8.0%	7.50
Burgundy	12.5%	5.50
Pinot Noir	13.7%	3.80
Moscato	11.0%	10.50
White Grenache	10.5%	7.00
Chablis	10.2%	5.00
Sangria	7-10%	3.80
Skinnygirl Sangria	10.5%	3.30

Liquor and Mixed Drinks

Alcohol always has calories, but we are counting carbs not calories. Still it helps to understand a few things about alcohol when it comes to calories and carb-counting.

Pure alcohol is high in calories. Everclear 190 proof which is 95% alcohol has 226 calories in 1.5 ounces; the rest is water. There are no carbs in it.

Alcohol is made by fermentation, which is a process where Yeast eats up sugars and turns them into alcohol. To make alcohol, you start with sugars which are a type of carbohydrate. These sugars in beers and wines are mostly from either grapes or barley. Vodka is made from potatoes; tequila is made from blue agave, rum from sugar cane, and other liquor from a number of plants.

The carbs are created by the way alcohol is made. If the yeast isn't 100% effective at converting all the sugars to alcohol, there will be sugars left over in the beverage resulting in a more caloric drink and this also creates unique flavors. Drinks that are more flavorful will usually have more calories per unit of alcohol. Not to worry, for there are many choices of flavors that have very low carb content. A drink with less alcohol tends to be not as sweet. Your body tends to burn up alcohol calories before it burns up food calories. If you are not on a low carb diet, the carbs start being burned up right after the alcohol calories. Being a low-carb diet reduces fat storage while it burns fat calories for fuel.

Since these alcohol calories being the first priority, there can be a tendency to speed up the buzz from drinking. For most people, this means you get the same buzz on less alcohol. Low-carb drinking often has a lower ABV (alcohol by content) but the drinker gets the effects of alcohol faster. A similar effect is what happens when you drink on an empty stomach. So if you are on keto and drinking on an empty stomach, beware that you will probably get inebriated faster than usual.

A rum with a Diet Coke will get you more buzz than a low-carb beer. Rum and Diet Coke has no carbs. Straight hard alcohol, including vodka, gin, rum, tequila, and whiskey has zero grams of carbs or sugar per ounce.

Bicardi flavored rums are generally 35% alcohol (70 proof) and have about 4g of carbs per shot (1.5 oz.) Flavored vodka's are a favorite of keto-drinkers.

Flavored vodka usually has zero carbs, but don't confuse this flavored vodka with vodka drinks which often have sweet flavorings that contain carbs. In terms of "buzz per carb," the flavored vodkas take first place. FYI: Champagne has about 1.6 carbs in each 4 oz. serving, very low.

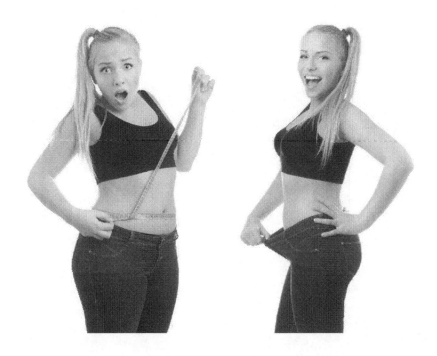

CHAPTER 7: THROW AWAY YOUR FOOD SCALES

You may need to unlearn a few things.

Now that you are on keto, you can fry foods in vegetable oil, canola oil, peanut oil, almost any kind of oil. You can soak your entrees in butter with zero guilt. Fat is good, so long as it's not around your hips and ass. It does seem strange after being taught all your life that fat is the enemy. You are starving your body of carbs and your body will eat what is left for it, the fat! Since your body is devouring fat now, it's ok to eat the stuff - in fact it's good.

For years the phrase *portion control* was drilled into everyone's head as a singular pinnacle of eating properly. We were told without portion control, all diet efforts will be futile. We were taught and drilled on portion control as being the key to dieting of all kinds. Well, now you can forget that, and I'm going to show you a quick and sure way to know exactly how to measure your food.

A lot of all the portion control talk was incorporated into diet *sales* literature. You order pre-measured meals to save time, for accuracy, to make sure you don't over-eat. If you believed that if you ate five ounces instead of four ounces of broccoli, you would ruin your diet, then you've taken the sucker bet. It just isn't true. Millions of meals have been measured to make sure nobody had 4.25 ounces of chicken instead of the prescribed 4.0 ounces. Nobody gets fat eating a quarter of an ounce of chicken. They get fat when they eat brownies when nobody's watching, not because they had too much chicken.

Remember, instead of a brownie, have a nice glass of Chablis. A two-inch square brownie with icing is about 14g of carbs. A 3.5 ounce glass of Chablis is only 2.6 carbs, so pour yourself a double and you are still not overindulging.

The trick to staying on keto is making these little deals along the way that keep you happy and satisfied. You eat smarter.

Question for you? Can you visualize how what four ounces (weight) of cooked green beans looks like?

Answer:

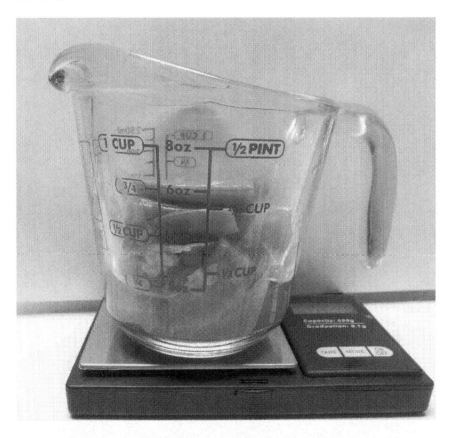

Here's why you do not need food scales: To portion your vegetables, simply consider all portions to be by volume one-cup.

One cup of peas and carrots is about 4 ounces.

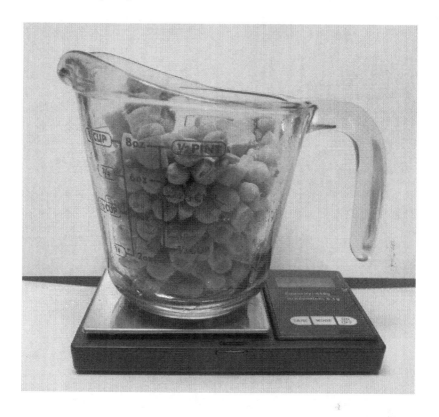

The only tool you need to stay on Keto is one measuring cup, or just cup your two hands to measure one cup. Look again at the chart with vegetable carb values. Simply consider one-cup, which is by weight about 4 ounces as a suitable amount of allowed vegetables. This approximation works just great and save a lot of time and worry. You are not going to suddenly fall out of ketosis by eating two extra spoonful's of a vegetable. Sorry, but you will rarely be eating bread and potatoes except on your birthday but you will be able to get a buzz on and lose weight. It's a choice.

One cup of broccoli = 4 ounces weight

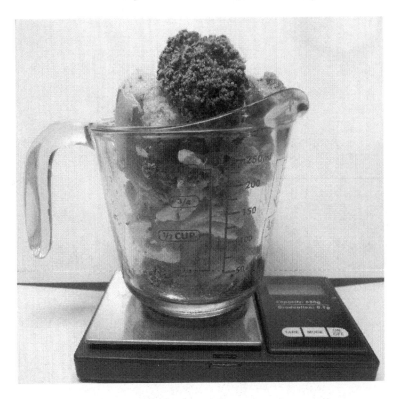

Faux Mashed Potatoes:

An entire head of cauliflower is about 27 grams of carbohydrates. Just trim the green off, boil it about 20 minutes or until very soft, then add a tiny bit of milk, perhaps some salt, pepper, and powered garlic, and puts lots of butter in it. Voila! You have fake mashed potatoes. The first time I made this dish, I grilled a ribeye to go with it. I was craving a nice grilled steak and mashed potatoes, and this is a pretty close substitute.

One cup of whole milk has about 12g of carbs. Just so you know, skim milk and low fat milk ALL have about 12 grams of carbs. So you can eat a half head of mashed cauliflower that includes a quarter cup of milk and it all adds up to about 20 carbs.

One medium yellow squash = 4 ounces weight

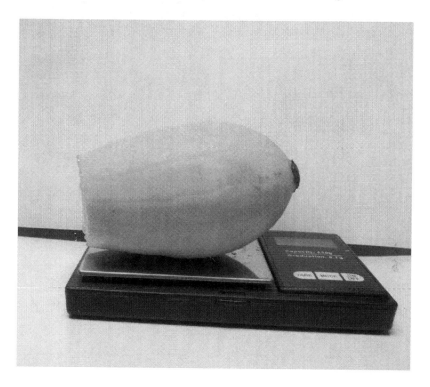

A favorite dish of keto-eaters is sweet onions and yellow squash. A cup of squash and onions pan-fried in oil is only about 10g of carbs. This is a tasty dish and easily manageable.

Remember, on keto you can eat butter and oil of just about all kinds. I fry chicken with a flour-egg batter and cook in vegetable oil, peanut oil, or olive oil and an entire fried battered breast is just 10 g of carbs.

After you are on keto for a month, you will notice your appetite diminishes. For some people it only takes two weeks or so. My advice is try hard to get past that first two weeks or month. Things will get a lot easier, I promise.

Vegetable	Carbs g per Cup / 4 oz weight
Zuchinni / yellow squash	6g / 7g
Green Peas	16
Carrots	7
Broccoli	6
Green beans	7
Asparagus	5
Bell peppers	6
Mushrooms	2.3
Spinach	7
Avocados	12
Cauliflower	5
Lettuce	1
Garlic	1 per clove
Cucumbers	3
Brussel Spouts	8
Celery	med stalk 1.2g
Tomatoes	1 medium red 5g
Radishes	10 radishes = 1 g
Onions	half cup 6g
Eggplant	4.8
Cabbage	5
Artichokes	13
Turnips	8
Beets	13
Potato	37
Sweet Potato	24
Mashed Potato	32
French Fries	48
Corn (cup) / one ear	31 / 17
Onion Rings	27

CHAPTER 8: WE'VE GOT THE MEATS

Jersey Shore's Vinny Guadagnino– is a huge keto dieter. He gets about 80 percent of daily calories from fat, 20 percent from protein, and 10 percent from carbohydrates. Your body is a powerful and smart furnace that will burn fat for fuel.

Choosing the meats you eat is about 90% of planning a keto diet and there are hundreds of delicious choices. Remember that bacon and cheese are 'free', so you can skewer chicken and bacon and outdoor grilling is very tasty. Try wrapping bacon around asparagus to go on the grill. Weave in some bell peppers and onions on the skewers for a variation of a keto healthy snack. Or you can use slices of zucchini and cherry tomatoes (6 of the cherry tomatoes are only 6 carbs.)

Meat is a complete, high-quality protein containing all of the essential amino acids the body needs for optimal health.

Most meats have about 25 grams of protein per 3 ounces. Dairy has 8g protein per cup, eggs 6g of protein each, and vegetables or nuts are about 2 to 5 g of protein. Meat is the natural source for vitamin B12. B12 is also known as cobalamin; it's water-soluble, and in the metabolism of every single cell in your body and also a cofactor in DNA synthesis in both fatty acid and amino acid metabolism.

New research challenges the widespread belief that white meat, such as chicken, is better for cholesterol levels than red meat, such as beef, pork, or lamb. Recent studies suggest that cholesterol is about the same in each of them.

MEATS	
Ribeye steak	0
Sirloin	0
Brisket	0
Fried Chicken Breast batter fried	9
Fried Pork Chops med/lge	7 to 10
Pulled Pork	0
Rotisserie Chicken whole chicken	6
Meatloaf	2.3
Grilled Wings	7
Fried Wings flour-coated w/skin	0.8
Chicken Nugget (1) McDonalds	2.8g
Chicken Tenders (4 pcs)	10
Chicken Strips Grilled	2
Roasted Pork tenderloin	0
Terriaki Chicken (6 oz)	8
Pork ribs babyback half rack/ full rack	2g / 4g
Shrimp Fried battered fried	1.29
Shrimp Grilled skewer (4 med pcs)	1
Fish fillet batter-fried	17
Scallops batter-fried	1.68
Flounder grilled / batter-fried	11.4
Hamburger 1/2 lb. (80/20)	0
Sausage patty	3.3
Bacon per slice	0.1
Deli chicken or ham (one slice)	1.19

When you eat BBQ, whether at home or dining out, the source of carbs is the sauces and sometimes filler. An entire rack of baby back ribs has only 4g of carbs but sauces are often packed with sugar. The average BBQ sauce is very high in carbs, often about 7g of carbs per tablespoon. This doesn't mean you can't have sauces and condiments, you just have to be sure and count them and use them sparingly. Both hickory smoked BBQ sauce and the Carolina tangy have 7g per tablespoon. The BBQ sauce is not terrible for you at all, you just have to use it sparingly. For example: Eat a rack of babybacks or spareribs and rub them in two tablespoons of sauce, salt and pepper and the total carb content is 4 + 14 = 18g of carbs. Even with a third tablespoon of sauce, the total is only 25g of carbs. That is close to your daily limit if you try to keep it under 35 to 40 g per day, but it is quite doable and delicious.

A teaspoon of Worcestershire sauce is 1.1g carbs.
Catsup is normally about 27% sugar and one teaspoon will set you back 4.5g carbs. Personally, I don't eat the catsup because there is so much more flavor in a good BBQ sauce with much lower carb content. Learn to 'spend' your carb allowances on items with good flavor that help curb your appetite. Next time you shop at the grocery store, check out some of the low sugar and non-sugar BBQ sauces.

You can also try making your own carb-free BBQ sauce. Make enough to fill a bottle and keep it on hand as a very low-carb condiment to have handy.

Ingredients

2 1/2 6-oz cans Tomato paste.

1/2 cup Apple cider vinegar.

1/3 cup Splenda (or any sweetener of choice, preferably either powdered or liquid)

2 tbsp Worcestershire sauce *

1 tbsp Liquid hickory smoke.

2 tsp Smoked paprika.

1 tsp Garlic powder.

1/2 tsp Onion powder.

You can add water to make it a thin dipping sauce. This recipe makes about a pint (2 cups) of low-carb sauce. The 6 oz can of tomato paste has a total of 37 carbs. About a quarter cup of sauce will have around 9g of carbs, so don't think of this sauce as completely 'free', use it sparingly. A pinch of cayenne can make it hotter if that is your preference.

The Chicken Shrine

Every time I go to Wal-Mart or my Kroger store, I walk up to the heat-lamp kiosk and admire the carb-free rotisserie chickens and smoked ribs - all cooked that morning fresh. Millions of those delicious, juicy, glistening chickens are sold every day; America loves them and they are good, healthy, and low-cost items that play perfectly into the keto diet. Zero (count'em) zero carbs!

There is another indulgence I allow myself and it is another of those American-favorites: the batter-fried chicken tender. You have to be very careful with this one; each tender is 4 to 5 carbs. The over-zealous keto food cops will tell you to not eat these because they think of you as a child with no self-control at all. I have a theory that a lot of dieticians and so-called healthy cooks probably have little faith in mankind and they think we all have no self-control because we decided to go on a diet. I, on the other hand, think of the reader of this book as a reasonable, healthy adult who can make an intelligent decision and stick to it.

That said, if you are really hungry and want something good to eat while on the keto plan, get yourself 3 or 4 of these 5g carb chicken tenders. Total is about 20g of carbs, half of your daily allotment. Add in a cup of one of your favorite vegetables, and two glasses of white wine. The total of chicken tenders + veggie + 2 wines = 20g + 7g + 2 (3.5g) = about 34 g of carbs, still way under your daily max of 35 to 40g of carbs. You'll be eating great, maybe get a little buzz doing and still remain on your diet.

Remember, depending on a person size, age, and metabolism - many people will remain in ketosis by keeping carbs under 40 to 45 grams. If you eat 25g one day and 45 the next, it isn't the end of the world. Use your common sense. Before keto, you were likely eating 250 to 325 g of carb a day - and if you have 45g one day, it just isn't the end of the world. You have to be nice to yourself as you relearn how to eat in a healthy way.

One of the world's wealthiest men, Warren Buffett once put being healthy into a nice reasonable perspective. I'm paraphrasing here: "Imagine you are only allowed to buy one car, one automobile in your entire lifetime. You would take care of it because it is the only one you are every allowed to have. Treat your body the same way."

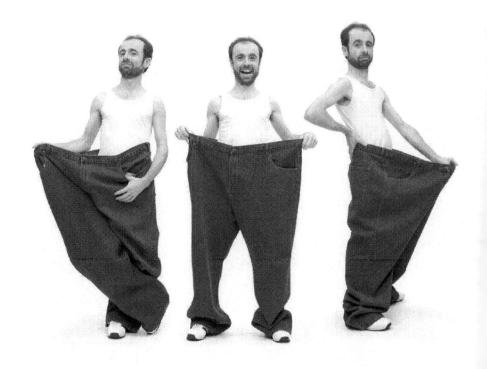

CHAPTER 9: THE MYTHICAL SUGAR MONSTER

Sugar is not the enemy. The problem with sugar is that we're eating so much of it. In 1700, when sugar was a rarity and only for the wealthy, average consumption was at approximately 4 pounds per year. Two-hundred years later by 1900 - that number had risen to 90 pounds per year. By 2008, more than half of Americans consume a half pound of sugar daily, a full 180 pounds of sugar per year.

From 4 pounds per year in 1700 to 180 pounds by 2008 - that's an increase of 45 times more sugar.

35% of the sugar we consume is converted to fat that can be converted to energy later. 50 percent of the sugar we consume today comes from high-fructose corn syrup in fat-free foods like salad dressings and regular soft drinks. It is ironic that fat-free foods we eat are loaded with sugar that converts directly to fat. That is how our intention to eat fat-free backfires on us - and the sellers of these products are not going to point that out to us. In this way, we are on our own.

These outrageous levels of sugar consumption are an enormous part of the health problem in North America today, quite directly responsible for obesity, diabetes, and a host of degenerative diseases. It isn't the sugar that is 'bad', it is the fact that the average consumption is so high. Anything to this sort of excess could be equally harmful. Though it is rare, there are people who have eaten so many carrots their skin turns yellow-orange. The fix is simple, stop eating so many carrots - and the body corrects the malfunction. The same type healing will happen by reducing the amount of sugar we eat. The amazing thing is just how very fast your body rebounds from excessive sugar intake. Even in one day, you feel a difference. For some people the transition is easy and for others more difficult. One thing that makes this drastic change easier to endure, is what you eat when you stop eating sugar. High fat and low carb intake - counters the effect somewhat for most people. The good news is that in only four or five days, if you were consuming high amounts of sugar, the major part of the adjustment is over quickly.

CHAPTER 10: GET YOUR DOCTOR'S APPROVAL

Why get your doctor's approval?

You must be sure there is nothing specifically about your health that could be damaged by a keto diet. When I first considered keto, I was at my cardiologist for a routine checkup and tests. I knew I needed to lose weight so I asked if I could or should consider the ketosis diet. I was actually surprised at how fast and without any hesitation at all, my doctor said, "yes." He did not follow his comments with a list of things not to do. As part of my examination that day, I had routine bloodwork done. The results followed in a few days and I made a copy and printed it out, so I could have a baseline of my results. A few months later, after losing just over 30 pounds, I had bloodwork done again at my regular doctor and we compared the results with my 'before keto' numbers. My pre-keto results all had normal numbers and so did my during-keto numbers. A doctor might say it differently but I was glad to see that all my numbers were still within recommended ranges. I take blood pressure medicine every day, my meds were reduced after I lost weight and it turned out I was able to completely eliminate (per my doctor's instruction and approval) one of my medications.

The advice and opinions in this book are not a substitute for you talking to your physician. You must be totally responsible for your own health and there is better way than to coordinate with your medical professional that knows your conditions and history. Not doing so, you could unknowingly do yourself harm.

The keto diet has been shown to have many health benefits, including weight loss and possibly reducing the risk or severity of diseases such as type 2 diabetes and epilepsy. According to a study published in August 2013 the European Journal of Clinical Nutrition, there's also some evidence that the keto diet can help clear up the skin, because high-glycemic foods (high carb foods) can promote acne.

The Atkins diet has been around since the 1970's and it is the same as the keto diet except that it gradually reduces carbs and the body slowly enters ketosis after the first few weeks.

Benefits of Keto Diet

- Curbs appetite
- Lose more weight faster than low-fat diets
- Greater proportion of fat loss comes from you abdominal cavity
- Triglycerides tend to drop drastically (fat molecules in bloodstream)
- Increased levels of 'good' HDL cholesterol
- Reduced blood sugar and insulin levels
- Often lowers blood pressure
- Improved 'bad' LDL cholesterol levels

Since the keto diets often reduce your retention of fluids, you should be aware of this and you may find that you need to drink more water or other fluids. Also, many people switching to keto will be taking in less salt. Again, if you have personal concerns about these, you should consult your physician prior to going on keto. You need this peace of mind before you start.

CHAPTER 11: USE KETOSIS FOR HUNGER SUPPRESSION

Anyone who's lost weight on a diet initially but gained the weight back afterwards already understands that most diets are not sustainable. Most diets leave you feeling hungry and unsatisfied almost continuously. A ketogenic approach actually suppresses hunger and appetite – this can make it more effective for weight loss than other eating fads and diets. You can actually use ketosis for hunger suppression. Learn to use keto as a better method than regular diets to keep your body from screaming for something to eat all the time.

Ketosis Vs Traditional Dieting

Although ketosis can be achieved through intermittent fasting, this is not the form of the diet that has the most success. Merely switching to low carb intake while keeping your proteins about the same - will bring about ketosis for most people in only two to four days. This can be the beginning of the end of food cravings regularly throughout the day. You should know that ketosis and intermittent fasting are not the same and simply crashing your body into ketosis is not the way to easy appetite suppression. The ketogenic diet has a structure to follow. Between weeks one and two, you will likely experience a huge drop in hunger. Your body really can adapt this fast.

It is quite easy to binge eat without having the more chronic diagnosis of binge eating disorder (BED.) When our little binges become regular and severe, much like an alcoholic who hides behavior and often goes on benders of too much drink – then the diagnosis of BED applies. Most of us never go to this chronic stage, which can be life-threatening and requires professional medical treatment. On most diets, it is quite common for people to get so hungry and cravings so intense, that a few hours or a day of two of eating one's favorite indulgences is not uncommon at all. This is normally followed by guilt and then bargaining with oneself to get back on track and to try again. Keto actually changes the body chemistry in ways that other diet usually fail to do. Simply eating healthier is often just not enough to diminish appetite and it sometimes plays into creating a larger appetite than one had when beginning the diet. This is why the failure rate is so high with traditional dieting. When one follows a strict calorie-counting diet, perhaps even resorting to kits of pre-package food in portions – it can create a sort of psychological vacuum where the dieter feels out of control. This is the last feeling you want when entering a serious venture at losing weight.

I found that being able to drink alcohol in a normal manner while still sticking to a keto diet did a lot toward having me feel in control while changing my eating habits. Keto, unless it's the very strict sort of keto diet where foods are counted, weighted and vilified – is actually a very user-friendly way of eating. Going to a moderate keto diet does not require calorie counting, weighing food, or that you must think of food in some moral, 'good or bad' sense. You can let go of all that and still have a very successful experience on keto.

It's going to be different for each of us of course, but I felt in control of my eating at all times. Does this mean I could eat all and everything I could think of? Certainly not. But it did mean that on my worst day food cravings, I could have gone out and eaten a rack of ribs, a slice of Texas toast, and have three or four beers- and still stay on my diet. Funny thing, but even though I had that example 'ribs and beer' meal in my head, I never actually did go out and order it. Just knowing that I could have on any day I wanted, was enough for me to feel in control. There were days when I was hungry and I always keep a number of frozen ribeye steaks and packs of those steam vegetable foods stocked in my freezer. There were many days when I had a ribeye and these vegetables and they were enough to get me to a point of satiation without even coming close to going off the keto diet. The ribeye of course has zero carbs, and even a whole pack of those steamed veggies (broccoli, carrots, cauliflower are my favorite) was only about 15 carbs (two cups.)

So I have devised a few ways to reward myself. You should have a good stash of your favorite permissible foods around. Think of then as a special 'go to' when you need it. This has also helped me feel in control of my diet.

After you are in ketosis for a few weeks, it actually feels physically bad to binge. Once, when I was about two months into my keto eating, I made the mistake of going to the grocery store when I was extremely hungry. A box of my favorite devil's food donuts with chocolate icing came home with me. Within half an hour I had already eaten three of them. I almost got physically ill and a dull very uncomfortable feeling came over me. I had just bombed my system with carbs and sugar to the max. I only got to enjoy the donuts for about 15 minutes and then I felt really bad. I promised myself I would make a point to remember this, and I have.

Of course we all know it's just common-sense not to have a hidden store of Little Debbie's or our favorite chocolate chip cookies stashed in the pantry for emergencies. What I did do was to make sure I stocked up on some of my favorite dishes. Yours will be different than mine of course. I absolutely love a good pot-roast smothering in sweet onions and lots of natural juices for gravy. I cook my pot-roasts in the crock pot slow cooker on a bed of sliced onions, no spices but salt, pepper, and a splash of Worcestershire sauce. I always let it cook for an extra long time at least 8 hours but usually close to ten hours (on low.)

I found that my ribeye steaks and pot-roasts were tasty foods and I can eat as much as I want and still stay on my diet. When you have those kinds of meals available to you, you will rarely if ever feel you are not in control. Feeling in control is not something you usually associate with any diet, but on keto, I can do it.

Why Calorie Counting is Impractical

Short-term weight loss is pretty easy for most people. Any of us can follow a strict diet for a short period of time to shed pounds. Unfortunately, for most dieters that weight gradually comes back over time – and often leaves us weighing more than they did to begin with.

Keto is not a calorie-restrictive diet. Calorie-counting often ignores health and often leaves us with hunger pangs and food cravings, and often ignores nutritional safety.

One of the reasons that counting calories is so ineffective is that the body doesn't process all calories the same. Quality matters. Traditional diet foods, especially packaged foods, are not healthy for us and they certainly are not filling. Keto can be both healthy and filling - and it should be.

The focus becomes too much about how many calories you're eating and not enough about what the foods are doing for your body. Open pre-measured packets a few days and you will learn that they will not curb your cravings - and eating them day in and day out can be very demoralizing, counter-productive, and certainly not anything to look forward to the next meal, day after day. This is precisely why keto, I would say - increases your chances of success by ten-fold when compared to most diets.

Don't start your keto thinking is just another variant of a food fad diet; it isn't. What matters most for long-term health is being able to keep the weight off for good, so we need a way of eating that will be sustainable and not have our thoughts consumed with food all the time.

Over time, your body will adjust so you "eat to live", not "live to eat." This is a very comfortable feeling that many people never allow themselves to experience.

Hunger Suppression

Eating a typical low-carb (like Paleo or Atkins) has many benefits, but there's something special about the ketogenic diet and ketosis when it comes to weight loss and hunger suppression. That's because ketosis literally changes your metabolism so that the body begins breaking down fats for fuel instead of carbohydrates, producing ketone bodies as fatty acids that are broken down.

There is an experience that we've all had that can prove to you that keto suppresses appetite. Is it not true that just hours after we binge on carbs and sugars, we wind up craving them just as much again and again? This is because you gave your body what it wanted and in short order, like a two-year-old's-temper-tantrum is back again just demanding more. In keto - as soon as your body starts 'living off fats' instead of carbs, those monotonous demands by your body for more sugar and more carbs simply diminish! It's true. You are not depriving your body of anything; you are merely re-training it. You might find yourself craving a pot roast or a ribeye, and eating those things is perfectly ok because you stay in ketosis. In ketosis your cravings are *naturally* reduced – and so are cravings for foods that typically lead to overeating. When you go into ketosis, you are actually using your own body chemistry to curb cravings for sugar and carbs. *Keto is the diet that gets easier instead of harder.*

When carb intake is drastically reduced and fats are high, this causes the body to turn to fat for its fuel source instead of using carbs (glycogen) as it would otherwise.

Your body will produce fewer hormones (Ghrelin) that increase appetite and increase other hormones (such as cholecystokinin) that can make you feel full and satisfied. Ketones also appear to have a positive effect on leptin signals and the brain's hypothalamus region, which can prevent the slowing of our metabolism like what happens in other diets. Traditional diets, the ones that count calories and reduce intake send signals to the body that all these things need replacing (aka: appetite.) Ketones are beneficial for the brain, heart, and other muscle tissues of our bodies because they allow them to conserve blood sugar while using ketones for energy instead.

Many people on keto will experience an improvement in mental clarity, a higher energy level, fewer mood swings, and gain the ability to stick to the diet over time.

Eating high-quality dense foods instead of cutting off and reducing good foods - naturally diminishes our appetite. You are simply giving your body plenty of healthy foods that it naturally craves. Our bodies naturally burn through carbohydrates first, so it doesn't take long for the body to send signals, it needs more of the stuff.

Many diabetics eat a diet similar to keto because these diets help prevent large swings in blood sugar. Intense swings in blood sugar trigger appetite signals and food cravings. This is a terrific benefit of the keto diet.

CHAPTER 12: MAKING YOUR HOME KETO FRIENDLY

I hope by now you realize that you can still drink, be on a healthy diet - and enjoy appetite suppression all at the same time.

Making your home and kitchen keto-friendly will help you become successful at dropping the pounds. Keto is the only diet or eating plan that after the first 30 days, I actually wanted to continue the plan, instead of starting to count the days until it's over.

Another nice and encouraging thing about keto is that you will drop some weight almost immediately - most people after only four or five days and into the second and third week experience a very noticeable weight loss. Actors and fighters use low carb / no carb plans to reduce weight quickly; it is one of the most effective diets to do that.

I don't need to name all the things you should not have available, you already know. Get rid of the sugars and carbs. I know of one lady who went keto and she had teenagers in the house. When they threatened mutiny if she got rid of their snacks, they found an unusual compromise. Her kids agreed to keep all the sugar and carbs in their rooms. You won't have to go to that extreme, but you do need to place all the temptations out of sight and out of mind.

When you go shopping buy the right foods. Get a variety, so you can always find something that suits your appetite. Make a list. Get a three to five day supply of your favorite foods that you can eat on keto. (It was ribeye steaks and pot roast for me with good vegetable steam packs.) Some people do better If they have hot meals with good portions, rather than trying to eat cold nibbles of diet food. Keto offers you what few diets do. Since you are not counting calories, you can prepare delicious hot meals with generous portions and stay well within your low-carb goal. When you get hungry, eat. Keto doesn't have to limit your food; the goal of keto is to change the way your body metabolizes food. You body's engine will be running off of fat mostly, burning it up every minute of every day and night - even while you sleep.

When you first start keto, you need to be aware of the contents of all the foods you take in. At first, you might have to do a lot of nutritional label content reading, but soon you will figure out and have experience to know exactly what you can eat.

Peanut butter and ketchup have very high sugar contents. Ketchup is often up to 27% sugar. Two tablespoons of peanut butter contain about 7 grams of carbs and 4 grams of sugar, a cup of a fresh vegetable has about the same amount of carbs but no sugar at all. You'll be surprised how fast you learn a few simple things about your food selections. It is actually much easier than you might think; this is part of the beauty of the keto diet.

Use your common-sense. There is nothing 'wrong' about using a dollop of ketchup once in a while to get a taste you desire or like. For some reason, nutritionist and also some of your friends who may have appointed themselves as keto-cops just love to preach their own gospel about 'bad foods.' But the truth is, you are an adult and do not deserved to be talked to like a child. A teaspoon of ketchup contains about 1.5 g of carbs and it won't matter if you have 30 carbs or 31.5 carbs on any particular day, you are still keeping them low enough for a good stable keto diet. When one of the 'self-appointed keto-cops' calls me out for salting my food or using a tablespoon of ketchup, I have to call BS on them. It was Mark Twain said that, "You shouldn't get into an argument with a stupid person, because onlookers usually can't tell which one of you is stupid, and it might make you look bad." My advice to you is count your own carbs and pick your battles.

I'm saying you don't have to go through your pantry and throw out all the condiments, you only have to be mindful of what you eat. And sorry, if you dip into the peanut butter jar five times a day while nobody's looking, you probably need to get rid of it.

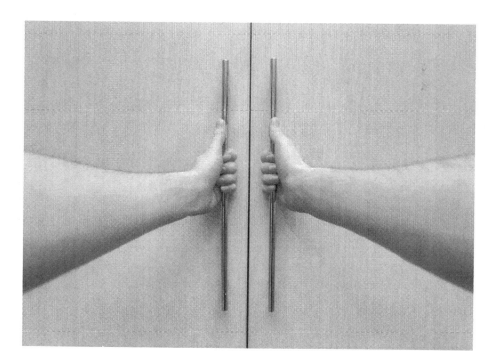

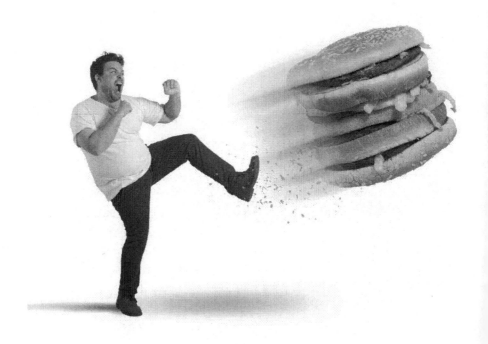

CHAPTER 13: KETO EXTRAS

It Can Get You Out Of A Weight-Loss Plateau

If you're currently experiencing a weight-loss plateau where your current meal plan or diet just doesn't seem to be effective anymore, this might be the time to try something different, like the keto diet.

The keto diet increases fat burn by putting your body in a state similar to fasting. Your body begins to use the fat it stored as a direct source of energy and by doing this, your body goes into a higher level of fat-burning. This can be reinvigorating in so many ways, and motivating as you start to lose the pounds you've been trying hard to shed.

It May Regulate Your Hormones

Interestingly enough, with the keto diet increase of ketones in the body, studies have shown a beneficial impact on regulating the hormones that affect your appetite. After eating, the hormone called cholecystokinin (CCK) is released by your intestines. That CCK hormone is responsible for stimulating the digestion of fats and proteins, and can delay the emptying of the stomach which reduces appetite. This means your hormones are actually helping to regulate food intake. Talk to your doctor always to be sure you do no harm to your body.

It Can Make You More Focused

Ever experienced "brain fog?" Improper diets often lead to challenges with mental sharpness and focus. The good news is, with the ketogenic diet's origins being an aid for children with epilepsy, it's no surprise that the diet has shown benefits to brain function.

When the body is in a state of ketosis, the liver is producing more ketone bodies. It provides the brain with an energy source from fat which allows the brain to properly convert glutamate into GABA. This may keep dieters out of the brain fog caused by over-stimulation, and in a refined state of focus and clarity.

Improve Memory

When the keto diet was given to those in early stages of Alzheimer's disease, studies showed they experienced a greater improvement on memory. This occurs when the ketones in the body produced by the liver, reduce the free radicals in the brain causing it to function more effectively.

As age begins to take its toll on one's memory, it becomes increasingly important to essentially "feed the brain" what it needs. This is very in line with the keto diet, since the diet itself requires a steady intake of healthy fats, essential to brain function.

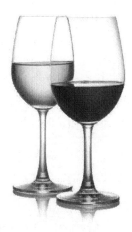

CHAPTER 14: NUTS

Pecans

Pecans are healthy nuts that provide a host of nutritional benefits.

They're not only low in carbs and high in fiber but also loaded with important nutrients like thiamine (vitamin B1), magnesium, phosphorus and zinc.

Total carbs per 1-ounce: 4 grams

Macadamia Nuts

Macadamia nuts are low-carb, high-fat nuts that are well suited for low-carb meal plans. They're an excellent source of B vitamins, magnesium, iron, copper and manganese (6).

Total carbs per 1-ounce: 4 grams

Brazil Nuts

Brazil nuts are large, low-carb nuts that are loaded with important nutrients. They're renowned for their high concentration of selenium. Just one Brazil nut delivers over 100% of the Reference Daily Intake (RDI.)

Total carbs per 1-ounce: 3 grams

Walnuts

Walnuts are not only low in carbs but also loaded with nutrients, B vitamins, iron, magnesium, zinc, polyphenol antioxidants and fiber. Walnuts contain healthy fats, including a plant source of omega-3 fats called alpha-linolenic acid (ALA). Diets high in ALA-rich foods have been found to reduce the risk of heart disease and stroke.

Total carbs per 1-ounce: 4 grams

Hazelnuts

Hazelnuts are rich in healthy fats, fiber, vitamin E, manganese and vitamin K. They also contain numerous antioxidants which help fight inflammation in your body. They are high in L-arginine, an amino acid that is a precursor to nitric oxide. Nitric oxide is a neurotransmitter that helps blood vessels relax and is important for heart health.

Total carbs per 1-ounce serving: 5 grams

Pine Nuts

Pine nuts have a distinct flavor and buttery texture due to their high oil content.They're particularly high in vitamin E, manganese, magnesium, vitamin K, zinc, copper and phosphorus.

Total carbs per 1-ounce: 4 grams

Peanuts

Though peanuts are technically legumes, they're commonly considered nuts and enjoyed the same way. Peanuts contain a wide array of nutrients, including folate, vitamin E, magnesium, phosphorus, zinc and copper. They're also high in protein; a 1-ounce serving has 7 grams. They are rich in antioxidants, including resveratrol, a phenolic antioxidant that has been shown to have protective effects against heart disease, certain cancers and cognitive decline.

Total carbs per 1-ounce: 6 grams

Almonds

These low-carb nuts are packed with nutrition. They're an excellent source of vitamin E, magnesium, riboflavin, copper, phosphorus and manganese). Almonds also happen to be particularly high in protein – delivering 6 grams per 1-ounce.

Total carbs per 1-ounce: 6 grams

Nut Butters

Natural Peanut Butter

Total carbs per 1-ounce: 5 grams

Regular Peanut butter carbs per 1-ounce: 6 grams

Almond Butter

Total carbs per 1-ounce: 6 grams

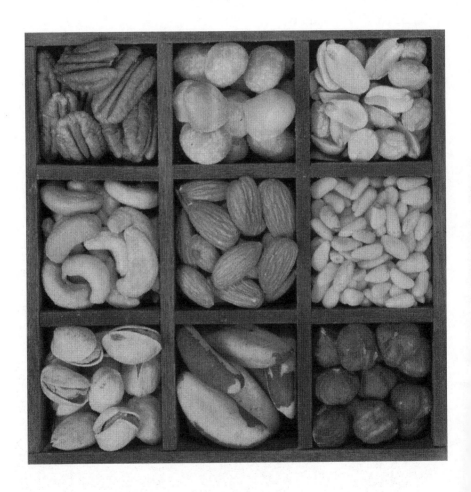

CHAPTER 15: AVOIDING LOW-CARB MISTAKES

Low-carb diets are very popular but it's also easy to make mistakes that can set you back. Here are some ideas around many stumbling blocks that can reduce the speed and success of your keto diet. Here's are some common mistakes:

Being Afraid of Eating Fat

This hint is about un-learning. Most people get the majority of their calories from dietary carbs – especially sugars and grains. When you remove this energy from your diet, you must replace it with something else - and that will be fat.

It is a mistake to think that cutting out fats on a low-carb diet will make your diet even healthier. It won't. In fact, it can work against you. Keto is all about maintaining a balance of nutrients. As you reduce carbs by 90%, you have to add fats to your diet. Failing to add fats to compensate could actually lead to an *increased appetite and eventually poor nutrition*.

A fat intake around 70% of total calories may is usually a good choice for some people on low-carb or ketogenic diets. To get fat into this range, you will have to choose fatty cuts of meat (ribeyes) and it's what you need to do.

Overeating Carbs:

While there is no strict definition of a low-carb diet, anything under 100-150 grams per day is generally considered low-carb. This amount is definitely a lot less than the standard Western diet.

 But if you want to get into ketosis – which is essential for a ketogenic diet – then this level of intake may be excessive.

Most people will need to go under 50 grams per day to reach ketosis. This doesn't leave a mountain of carb options – except vegetables and small amounts of berries and nuts - and your drinks of course.

If you want to get into ketosis and reap the full metabolic benefits of low-carb diets, going under 50 grams of will be necessary. My experience was reducing to between 30 and 40 grams of carbs a day was plenty to get the results I wanted.

Just so you know: When doctors are asked how many carbs for a keto diet, the recommendations are often much lower than most people would need. They make statements like, "20 grams a day is low enough to put almost anybody into ketosis." That is definitely not the same as saying that a low of 20 carb is necessary.

Quitting Too Soon

Your body is designed to preferentially burn carbs. Therefore, if carbs are always available, that's what your body uses for energy. On a keto diet you reduce carbs down so low that you cannot live off of them. This forces your body to shift into burning fat. And all of the fat will come from one of two places, you diet or your body's stores (the fat you want to lose.)

It only takes few days for your body to adapt to burning primarily fat instead of carbs; usually two to four days. After you get over the first four days or so, you are on your target.

Don't make the mistake of thinking that being on keto will feel like this the entire time; it won't. You'll get over it

Too Much Protein

Protein is a very important macronutrient and when people go on various diets, they often don't get enough protein. Since keto requires eating a lot of meats with fat, it is possible to eat too many proteins a day. Protein intake should be around 20 to 23% of caloric intake. Since meats have no carbs, you will probably be eating a lot of it but don't think you must eat only a small amount.

One of the major reasons keto can reduce appetite is that the protein actually improve feelings of fullness and it enhances the body's ability to burn fat burning better. Generally speaking, more protein should lead to weight loss and improved body composition.

However, low-carb dieters who eat a lot of lean animal foods can end up eating too much of it. Unlike you may have been taught, the fat you eat on keto is good for you. Your body is going to start processing these fats instead of carbs. These fats have to be available.

Eating far more protein than your body needs can result in some of its amino acids will being turned into glucose via a process called gluconeogenesis. It is possible that too much protein can actually prevent your body from doing to a full state of ketosis.

Not Replenishing Sodium

One of the main mechanisms behind low-carb diets is a reduction in insulin levels. In the body, insulin informs your fat cells to store fat and your kidneys to retain salt. On a keto diet insulin levels go down and your body starts shedding excess sodium – and water along with it. This is why people often get rid of excess bloating within a few days of low-carb eating. Low sodium levels can become problematic when your kidneys dump too much of it.

Some people on keto diets ignore this fact and can develop side-effects such as lightheadedness, fatigue, headaches, and even constipation. This can almost always be avoided by making sure you get plenty of salt and water. You may need to salt your foods if you haven't been doing so. Drinking a cup of broth can replentish salt in the body.

Not getting enough salt and water can increase your appetite and even cause other side effects.

Exercise

The keto diet plan does not require a regular exercise regimen. Sure, we all should get exercise in moderation. We all have our excuses for not getting enough exercise. Just moving around -, especially if you are older - keeps good health and flexibility and generates chemicals in the body that support a feeling of well-being.

For most people, losing weight on keto does not require a change in exercise regimen. For me, after I lost the first 20 pounds, with almost no exercise, I actually felt like getting out for a daily walk since my energy level was higher. Also losing a gut stomach and waistline was an incentive for me to add regular moderate walks to my daily routine. Doing so, made me feel even better in many, many ways. And just that little bit of exercise got me off a plateau weight that I was stuck on for almost two weeks. Try it!

Speaking of hitting those plateaus of weight, those are things experienced on almost all diets. Don't get discouraged if you plateau for a week or two at a time, just be glad you are not putting those pounds back on, and know that your progress will continue. You also have to stay honest with yourself; if you are eating 60 carbs a day instead of 25 to 45, that is probably the reason for your plateau. If you try various levels of carbs, give each of your test periods at least five to ten days to gauge results.

To the Reader: Good luck on your keto journey. I wish you all the best. IF YOU WOULD LIKE TO RECEIVE A FREE BONUS CHAPTER WITH FOOD CARB CHARTS TO PRINTOUT AND ALSO SOME GREAT LINKS TO KETO RECIPIES - ALL FREE

JUST SEND AN EMAIL WITH "KETO" IN THE SUBJECT LINE TO THIS EMAIL ADDRESS:

Apple@WriteThisDown.com   Be sure to put KETO in the subject line. And send me a note about your keto progress; I'd love to hear from you. - Art Mawkin